Tennis Ball Self-Massage

Effective Trigger Point Therapy to Relieve
Your Muscle and Joint Pain

Angie Sage

ISBN-10: 1533272603
ISBN-13: 978-1533272607

DEDICATION

This book is dedicated to those in search of their very own massage buddy without having to spend much money.

CONTENTS

INTRODUCTION

Do you ever have really stressful days that make you long for a good massage? Do you constantly wish to visit a spa but simply never have the time? Do you know someone who gives great massages but he/she is simply nowhere to be found on that crucial moment when you need it?

There is a way for you to have your very own massage buddy without having to spend much money. Furthermore, this massage buddy can please you at any time and any place that you wish. If you are thinking that this is exactly what you need, maybe it's time that you consider doing a tennis ball self-massage! All you need is a tennis ball and you can massage all the aches away!

CHAPTER 1 - WHAT IS TENNIS BALL SELF-MASSAGE?

Do you ever have really stressful days that make you long for a good massage? Do you constantly wish to visit a spa but simply never have the time? Do you know someone who gives great massages but he/she is simply nowhere to be found on that crucial moment when you need it? There is a way for you to have your very own massage buddy without having to spend much money. Furthermore, this massage buddy can please you at any time and any place that you wish. If you are thinking that this is exactly what you need, maybe it's time that you consider doing a tennis ball self-massage! All you need is a tennis ball and you can massage all the aches away.

Massage refers to the manual manipulation of body tissues. This involves applying pressure on the different parts of the body – stationary or moving – to enhance relaxation, health and well-being. It can be done manually or with the use of a massaging device. You see, there are different ways to apply pressure on your body. You can use your hands, your fingers, your elbows, your knees, your forearms, or even your feet. Some people use electric massaging devices, others use manual massaging devices, and some people like to get creative and grab random objects around them which they can use to apply pressure on their body. It can be a stick, a bottle, or a ball. There are endless possibilities.

Now, are you wondering how a tennis ball can help ease your sore muscles? A tennis ball massage is an innovative massage method. Basically, the idea is to put the ball between your body and another object - this can be the floor or the wall among other things – and to push your body against it, gradually applying pressure and pressing on sore spots. A lot of people who opt to try this do so because one can use it for a self-massage and unlike electric massage devices a tennis ball is fairly cheap. Furthermore, the ball is small enough to fit in your bag or purse, and so you can take it with you all the time, allowing you to do a self-massage anytime and anywhere that you need it. So take that, it's a cheap yet very effective way to get rid of sore muscles.

Let's start with the basics. If you are planning to try the tennis ball self-massage, the first thing that you'll need is of course a tennis ball. Maybe you can get two or three just to be sure. Next, find a flat and hard surface you can lie on. If you're uncomfortable on the bare floor, you can always use a carpet, a yoga mat or any exercise mat. In some variations of the tennis ball self-massage you may lean on the wall instead of lying on the floor. Go ahead and look around your house! Move some furniture around if you need to and make sure that you have a decent space on the wall where you can lean on. Finally, figure out which part of your body you wish to massage. There are other things that you can utilize along with the tennis ball, but we'll get to that later.

Trigger point or muscle knots refers to compressed muscle tissues. These commonly cause aches and pain in different parts of the body. Applying pressure on common trigger points in the head, neck, back, etc. can give you a great deal of satisfaction as these are usually the sweet spots of massage therapy. But how do these trigger points occur? Your muscle may contract when it is overloaded. This can be due to a physical trauma or an injury, repetitive stress on the muscle, or sudden muscle movements. Trigger points usually occur in similar areas, and so, in tennis ball self-massage, you can take advantage of these trigger points to get optimum results.

Angie Sage

CHAPTER 2 - TRIGGER POINT THERAPY FOR HEAD AND NECK

Headaches and neck pain are fairly common after a long day. Daily stressors like hunching over a computer and staying on your work desk all day may lead to the tightening of muscles in the upper shoulder and neck causing trigger points which result to painful muscle imbalance. This is where your tennis ball comes in! When you have headaches and neck pain, your "trapezius" and "levator scapula" muscles are inflamed. Therefore, these are the trigger points which you would like to target with your tennis ball.

How to Find the Trigger Points

Your "trapezius" muscle is easy to locate as it is a big muscle in your upper back. To find it, put your hands on your shoulders right at the side of your neck. That bulge that you are touching is the muscle you are looking for. Any muscle compression in the upper and middle part of your "trapezius" muscle may radiate up to your head, behind your skull, to your temples and behind your eyes, thus causing headaches and migraines.

The "levator scapula" muscle is the muscle that you use when you are elevating your shoulder blades. To find it, put your hands on both sides of your neck and feel for the spot where the muscles in your neck connects nicely with your shoulder blades. This is the spot that usually hurts when you are having a stiff neck.

Now that you have found the trigger points, it's time to massage yourself with your handy tennis ball! There are different techniques on how to use a tennis ball for self-massage depending on the area that you wish to massage. Go grab your ball and let's get started!

Massage to Relieve Headache (Trapezius Muscle)

1.   To target your "trapezius" muscle, first, lie down on the floor and relax.

2.   When you are ready, locate the bulge in your upper back and right beside your neck which we earlier identified as the trapezius muscle.

3.   Place your tennis ball under that area and slowly start moving your body, making small circles as you go.

4.   Push your body against the ball until you find the right pressure and gradually rotate and glide until you find sore points.

5.   Hold the ball under sore points for about 30 seconds or until you release the muscle knots.

6.   Just keep moving, gliding, rotating and sliding in all directions until you are completely satisfied.

That massage must feel great; you're off on a great start! Now, let's explore other ways to use a tennis ball for self-massage. In this next part, you will find instructions on different ways to massage the neck area.

Massaging the Neck (Levator Scapula)

1.   To massage your "levator scapula", recall the position of this muscle and try to locate where the muscle attaches to your shoulder blade. This is where you can usually find trigger points or muscle knots.

2.   Feel for the top inside part of your shoulder blade, this shall be your starting point.

3.   Put the tennis ball against the inside part of your shoulder blade.

4.   Remember your special spot on the wall? Go over there and lean against it, trapping the tennis ball between your shoulder blade and the wall.

5.   Start moving upwards and downwards. Nod your head as if saying "yes".

6.   Once you find a sore point, hold the ball over that spot for about 30 seconds or until you feel a release.
    There is another trick for dealing with neck pain using the almighty tennis ball which can be done by sitting on a relaxing chair.

Massaging the Neck (Levator Scapula) While Sitting on a Chair

1.   Find a chair that has a high headrest – one where you can rest your head on comfortably.

2.   Sit on your chosen chair and get comfortable.

3.   Put the ball between the side of your neck and the spine, just below your skull. This is your "levator scapula" muscle.

4.   Lean onto the ball against the chair and slowly nod up and down 10 times.

5.   When you are done, hold your position for about 1 minute.

6.   Pivot your head left and right. Repeat this 10 times.

7.   Ease into this position for another minute and feel your pain fade away.

If you feel like you need more magic, get two tennis balls – because we can't get enough of tennis balls – and try this massage technique using a sock.

Massaging the Neck (Levator Scapula) with Two Tennis Balls and a Sock

1.   Place two tennis balls inside a sock – please make sure the sock is washed and clean.

2.   Sit on a chair that has a high headrest and relax.

3.   Position your neck just between the tennis balls, make sure that your massaging tool is in contact with your "levator scapula" muscle.

4.   Once you are in position, gently nod your head up and down as if you're saying "yes". This should massage both sides of your neck nice and good.

5.   Repeat this motion up to 10 times and then hold the position for about 1 minute.

6.   After a minute, start pivoting your head left and right as if you're saying "no".

7.   Repeat this 10 times and then hold your position for a minute.

8.   Next, tilt your head to one side and start nodding up and down again.

9.   After about a minute, turn to the other side and do the same.

10.   Finally, face right and hold your head in that position for about a minute, then face front and then left doing exactly the same. Now that's oh so good!

Once you have released the compressions in your "trapezius" and "levator scapula" muscles, your headaches and neck pain should lessen if not totally disappear. And the best part is that you don't need to spend money on expensive massage spas! Your only tool, a tennis ball!

Angie Sage

CHAPTER 3 - TRIGGER POINT THERAPY FOR BACK, SHOULDER AND ARM

As mentioned in the first chapter, there are a number of common trigger points in your body. In this chapter, we will focus on releasing muscle compressions in the back, shoulder and arm areas.

The back, shoulder and arm muscles can easily be overworked as these are one of the most used muscle groups in your body. These are the muscles that support most of your movement and your posture. And so, if you feel sore in these areas, don't hesitate! Grab your tennis ball and give your muscles some love.

How to Find the Trigger Points

The lower part of your "travezius" muscle and your "levator scapula" muscle are also known as culprits for shoulder and back pain. Please refer to the first chapter to locate these trigger points.

Beside your spine and just below your "travezius" muscle, there are thick columns of muscles known as "rhomboids" – the muscle group has a rhombus shape, thus, the name - which are routinely filled with compressed muscles or muscle knots. These are common trigger points in the upper back, starting from the base of your neck all the way down to a spot just between your shoulder blades. As for the lower back, find a spot between your spine and your lowest rib. This trigger point is known as the "thoracolumbar corner". You will want to focus on this area if you are experiencing lower back pain.

Now, let's talk about shoulder pain. The trigger point in this area is tricky to find. However, do you want to know a secret? Find your shoulder blade and feel for a spot under the ridge bone. You can relieve shoulder pain by applying pressure nearly anywhere on this area. Other parts where trigger points can cause shoulder pain are along your rotator cuffs and your chest or pectoral region.

Aside from your back and shoulders, the muscles in your arms could also hold a good deal of tension. Arm pain can be attributed to a set of muscles attached to multiple ribs and located just underneath your shoulder blades. This muscle group is called the "serratus posterior superior" muscle. Muscle compressions in this area may refer pain or numbness to the upper arm and forearm. And since it's attached to the shoulder it may also cause deep aches in the shoulder.

Massaging the Travezius and Levator Scapula

If you think that the "travezius" and "levator scapula" muscles are responsible for your back pain or shoulder pain, please refer to the first chapter of this book for instructions on how to massage these trigger points.

Otherwise, please refer to the following massage techniques to address back, shoulder and arm pain.

Massaging the Back (Rhomboids and Thoracolumbar Corner)

For the rest of your back, we can use similar tennis ball self-massage techniques on the upper back and the lower back. Now, let's get creative!

1.   Find a clean sock and put two tennis balls inside.

2.   When you are ready, go to your special spot by the wall.

3.   Put your sock buddy against your back making sure that one ball is on either side of your spine and is pressing against the thick column of muscles there.

4.   Push against the wall and find the right pressure for your back.

5.   If you are focusing on your upper back:

a. Place the sock against your upper back, making sure that it is pressing against the "rhomboids".
b.   Roll down just until the tennis balls reach your lowest rib. Once there, slowly roll back up.
c. Find your soar points and focus on these spots for about 30 seconds or until you feel that your muscle knots are relieved.

6.   If it is your lower back that you wish to relieve:

a. Place the sock against your lower back just below your ribs. This is the spot where you can find your "thoracolumbar corner".

b.   Slowly roll down, stop just above your hip and roll back up.

c.Look for sore spots in your lower back and focus the pressure on these areas for about 30 seconds or until you are relieved.

7.   You may repeat the upper back and/or lower back tennis ball self-massage up to 8 times or until you are satisfied.

You may also do a variation of this massage by lying on the floor instead of pushing against the wall. You see, some people find it easier to apply just the right pressure against their back when they are pushing against the wall whereas some people feel that doing the tennis ball self-massage against the floor is fairly easier. Now, let's move on to shoulder blade massage.

Massaging the Shoulder Blade

1.   Lie down on the floor and place the tennis ball behind your shoulder blade.

2.   Relax, take a few deep breaths, and get rolling! Slide up, down, left or right.

3.   Feel free to explore this move while trying to find sore spots around your shoulder blade.

4.   Keep on massaging your shoulder for about 3 minutes or until you are satisfied.

You may also do a variation of this shoulder blade tennis ball self-massage against the wall. You see, other people find it easier to apply pressure on the shoulder blades by pushing against a wall. Try whatever works for you! Now, here are the steps on how to address pain in your rotator cuffs.

Massaging the Rotator Cuffs

1.   To access this area you need to get down on the floor and lie on your side.

2.   Bend your elbow at approximately 90 degrees.

3.   Once you are in position, put your tennis ball right outside your shoulder blade. Here, you will find your rotator cuff.

4.   Roll the ball around slowly, making small circles as you go.

5.   Feel for sore spots as you roll the tennis ball.

6.   If you feel like you found an area with compressed muscles, stop rolling the ball and focus the pressure on that area.

7.   Slowly stretch your arm, hold it for a count of 10 and then bend it back to its original position.

8.   Resume rolling the ball to look for sore spots and then do the same.

9.   Repeat this massage on your other arm.
   If your shoulder pain seems to be radiating from the front part of your shoulders, then it is possible that the muscle contractions occurred in your "pectoral region" or your chest area. Here's how you can massage your pectorals with a tennis ball.

Massaging the Chest or Pectoral Region

1.   To address pain in this area, you need to lie down on the floor face down.

2.   Put your tennis ball under your chest muscles and slowly start rolling.

3.   Gently explore this area until you find a sweet spot. Focus on this sore spot for a few minutes or until you feel a release.

Trigger points don't always occur in the spot where you feel the aches. Sometimes, the muscle compression occurs somewhere else and then it radiates pain to other parts of the body. This rule is true with arm pains as the sore spots usually occur in muscles from the shoulder or back area and then radiates the pain back to the arm. In the next massage, you will learn to address arm pain by massaging your "serratus posterior superior" muscle which can be found at your back, right beside the "rhomboids".

Massaging the Serratus Posterior Superior

1.   Lie on the floor facing up.

2.   Place a tennis ball against the upper right part of your back, a little to the right of the "rhomboids". (Please refer to chapter 3 for instructions on how to locate this muscle.)

3.   Lean against the ball until you are satisfied with the pressure.

4.   Slowly roll the ball to the right and then slowly roll back to your starting point.

5.   Look for sore spots and focus on these areas for about 30 seconds.

6.   Do this routine up to 8 times or until you feel satisfied.

7.   Repeat the massage against the upper left part of your back.

Now that's how you massage back, shoulder and arm pain away with the power of a tennis ball!

Angie Sage

CHAPTER 4 - TRIGGER POINT THERAPY FOR FOREARM AND HAND

Have you ever had persistent sores in your forearm and your hand that make finishing daily tasks harder than they already are? Did you ever have difficulty doing a plank while working out or difficulty carrying something because your hand hurts? Do you think the grip of your hand is getting weaker and are you having difficulty typing on a computer? Don't worry! There is a simple home remedy for that – a tennis ball!

In the previous chapters, you learned how to address pain in your head, neck, back shoulder and arm with the use of a tennis ball. Now let us discuss how to address pain in the forearm and hand. You see, in today's busy lifestyle, technology has high demands for the muscles in our hand. People spend hours typing in a computer, editing documents, browsing on the internet, thus overusing the muscles in their forearm and hand without even noticing it.

How to Find the Trigger Points

As mentioned in the previous chapter, muscle compressions in the "serratus posterior superior" muscle may also cause pain in the forearm. Please refer to chapter 3 for instructions on how to locate this muscle.

There is a think tendon at the back of your forearm consisting of all the muscles you can find just beyond your elbow. This is known as the "common extensor tendon". Muscle knots form in this area as a result of extensive use of fine motor skills, like when you use the computer all day or perhaps write a very long journal entry using a pen. Your hand may also have tight flexors due to overuse.

Massaging the Serratus Posterior Superior
If you think that the pain you're feeling is caused by compressions in this muscle, please refer to chapter 3 for instructions on how to massage this area.
For addressing pain in your forearm which is referred from trigger points in the "common extensor tendon" and hand pain caused by tight flexors, please refer to the following massage techniques.

Massaging the Forearm (Common Extensor Tendon)

Remember the technique where you put two tennis balls in a sock? You can use the same buddy for addressing pain in your forearm and wrist.

1.   Put two tennis balls in a sock.

2.   Place your massaging tool on top of a flat surface – preferably a table.

3.   Position your arm between the two tennis balls and

slowly start rolling back and forth.

4.   Cover your whole forearm, from the wrist, up until your elbow.

5.   Feel for sore spots and hold the pressure if you find any.

6.   Continue this routine up to 3 minutes or until you are satisfied.

Massaging the Hand

1.   Stand in front of a table and put the tennis ball on top of the table.

2.   Place the hand that you wish to massage on top of the ball.

3.   Put your other hand on top and gradually apply more pressure.

4.   Squeeze your ball by pushing your bodyweight against the table.

5.   Hold the pressure for about one minute.

6.   Roll the ball against your palm up and down, and then side to side.

7.   You may also try gliding the ball diagonally from left to right and then from right to left.

8.   Once you are satisfied, you may switch to your other hand and follow the same steps.

If you are more comfortable sitting on the floor or an exercise mat, feel free to do this hand massage on the floor.

Now that you know how to deal with trigger points in the forearm and hand, it would be a good idea to massage these spots at least once a day even if you don't feel pain. This way, the tendons in your forearm and hand would get stronger, thus preventing more serious injuries in the future.

CHAPTER 5 – TRIGGER POINT THERAPY FOR HIP, THIGH AND KNEE

Have you ever had difficulty sitting, standing and/or walking because of painful hips, thighs or knees? Do you hate having to stop and sit every now and then during walks at the mall, park, etc.? Well then, the next time that you experience aches in the hip, thigh or knee area, grab your tennis ball and roll the pain away!

How to Find the Trigger Points

If you are experiencing aches in the hip area, your "quadratus lumborum – small muscles in your lower back, tensor fascia latae – muscle attached above your hip joint, and piriformis – located in the buttocks" muscles are probably inflamed. These are the muscles that tend to radiate pain to your hips. Pain in this area may be caused by too much exercise, sitting too much, or wearing high heels for prolonged periods of time.

Pain in the thigh area is usually referred from the "quadriceps muscle". The quadriceps is a large group of muscles which covers the front of the upper leg or the thigh. This muscle group is used for walking, sitting, standing, bending, etc.

Knee pain is usually attributed to inflamed "quadriceps muscle". However, there is another muscle group that may cause pain in the knee area, the "hamstring". This is the set of muscles that you can find behind your thigh. It starts from the pelvis and crosses the hips and the knees.

Now, how do we address pain in the hip, thigh and knee areas? Here's how.

Massaging the Hip

1.   Lie down on the floor or on an exercise mat.
2.   Place the tennis ball beside your hip.
3.   Slowly lean on the tennis ball.
4.   Move your hip and leg as if you are making a circle with the ball. Repeat this about 10 times.
5.   Do the same on your other hip.

Massaging the Thigh and Knee (Quadriceps)

Aside from relieving aches in the thigh, this self-massage technique also helps in soothing muscle tightness in the hips and knees.

1.   Do a side sitting position on the floor or on an exercise mat.

2.   Place two tennis balls under the outer thigh of your right leg.

3.   Put your right arm in front of the balls for support.

4.   Slowly stretch your right leg out and then bring it back in. Do this about 10 to 20 times.

5.   Now, slide your thigh from left to right and vice versa so that the tennis balls would roll on the side of your thigh. Do this up to 2 minutes.

6.   Repeat the massage on the other thigh.

Massaging the Hamstring

1.   Sit on the floor.

2.   Put the tennis ball above your hamstring. This would be the part of your pelvis that you are sitting on.

3.   Place your hands beside your buttocks for support and push yourself off the floor.

4.   Move your hips from side to side so that the ball would roll across your hamstring muscles.

5.   Repeat this until you are satisfied.

6.   Move the tennis ball under your hamstring muscles just above the knee.

7.   Move your leg from left to right and vice versa so that the ball rolls across your hamstring muscles.

8.   Do the same on the other leg.

    This "hamstring" massage may be a little difficult because your arms will have to support your bodyweight, but the benefits are worth it! Now, remember the rule that the trigger point is not always located to the body part that hurts? This is true with pain in the knee area. To address pain here, you don't actually massage the knee. Methods include massaging the "quadriceps muscle" and the "hamstring" as instructed earlier in this chapter. If your knee still feels tight, try the following technique.

Massaging the Knee

1.   Sit on a flat surface. You may sit on the floor, on a stool, or on a chair.

2.   Bend one leg about 90 degrees.

3.   Place the tennis ball behind your knee, between your thigh and your leg.

4.   Hold your leg by the shin or by the ankle with both hands.

5.   Slowly squeeze the ball by pulling your leg closer to your body.

6.   Hold this position for 10 counts.

7.   Let go of the position and relax your knee for 10 counts.

8.   Pull on your leg again and hold for another 10 counts.

9.   Repeat this up to 8 times.

10.   Do the same on the other knee.

Congratulations! You now know a lot of basic techniques on how you can use a tennis ball as a handy massage tool. Always pack your new friend with you and say good bye to sore muscles as soon as you feel them.

Angie Sage

CHAPTER 6 – TRIGGER POINT THERAPY FOR LEG, ANKLE AND FOOT

Having aches in your leg, ankle or foot can be very excruciating! It's difficult to move around, it's difficult to walk, and it's difficult to focus. And so, learning some easy and cheap home remedies to address such aches could possibly save you from possible mishaps in the future like missing deadlines due to the agonizing pain, or not enjoying a party because you had to sit on the couch from start to finish.

How to Find the Trigger Points

Take a look at your legs and observe its shape at the back. The muscle that forms this area is called the "gastrocnemius muscle". Pain and aches in this area can be caused by walking, jogging, climbing, prolonged immobilization, etc. To find the trigger points here, look for the crease of your knee. Just below this you can find the upper medial trigger point and if you move down about an inch or two, there you will find the lower medial trigger point. Mirror this on the lateral side of your leg and you should find the upper lateral and lower lateral trigger points.

Pain in the ankle is usually referred from the "peroneus muscles" which can be found in the outer part of your lower leg. And so, to address aches in the ankle, you don't really massage the ankle itself. Remember, the spot that aches is not always the root of the problem.

Now, where does pain in the foot area root from? From your heel bone all the way to your toes there is a thick band of tissue known as the "plantar fascia". This can become inflamed due to overuse from workouts, stretching, excessive walking, etc. Thus, this is a good trigger point for addressing pain in the foot area.

Massaging the Leg

1.   Sit on a flat surface. An exercise mat or a yoga mat is highly recommended but not necessary.

2.   Stretch your legs out.

3.   Put the tennis ball underneath the part of your leg that you wish to massage. It is highly recommended that you focus on the trigger points referred to earlier in this chapter.

4.   Bend your other leg about 9o degrees, your foot should be flat on the floor.

5.   Place both of your hands behind you with elbows straight. This will serve as your support.

6.   Slowly slide your butt backward so that the ball would roll down your leg.

7.   Slide your butt forward so that the ball would roll up your leg.

8.   Continue the back and forth motion focusing on sore spots for about 20 seconds and then move the ball to another spot.

Massaging the Ankle (Peroneus Muscles)

1.   Sit on a flat surface. You can use a yoga mat or an exercise mat but it is not necessary.

2.   Stretch your legs out and twist one leg outward so that the peroneus muscles are facing the floor.

3.   Put the tennis ball underneath your lower leg.

4.   Bend your other leg about 9o degrees so that your foot is flat on the floor.

5.   Extend both of your arms and place them behind you for support.

6.   Now, scoot backward do that the ball would roll down your outer leg, feeling for sore spots along the way.

7.   Slide back up slowly so that the ball would roll up your outer leg, again, feeling for sore spots along the way.

8.   Repeat the back and forth motion until you are satisfied, focusing on sore spots for about 20 seconds.

Massaging the Foot (Plantar Fascia)

1.   Stand next to a wall or a chair for support. You can also do this sitting down

2.   Put the tennis ball on the floor.

3.   Place your foot on top of the ball so that it is directly under the arch of your foot and apply pressure by letting your weight sink in.

4.   Slowly move your foot from side to side so the ball would cross the arch of your foot. Repeat this for about one minute.

5.   This time, move your foot up and down so that the ball would roll from your heel all the way to your toe. Repeat this for about one minute.

Do the same on the other foot.

A FINAL WORD

I want to take this time out to thank you for purchasing this book! The next step is to take action on the advice you've just read about.

Please Leave a Review

Finally, if you enjoyed this book, please take the time to share your thoughts and post a review. It'd be greatly appreciated!

That review and feedback will help me improve the content in my books – and make each and every one more relevant and helpful to you.

Thank you again and good luck!

Angie Sage